This Tracker Belongs To:

_____

Week At A Glance

Abdominal Migraine

	1	2	3	4	5	6	7	8	9	10	11	12	13	14	15	16	17	18	19	20	21	22	23	24
S																								
M																								
T																								
W																								
T																								
F																								
S																								

Cyclic Vomiting

	1	2	3	4	5	6	7	8	9	10	11	12	13	14	15	16	17	18	19	20	21	22	23	24
S																								
M																								
T																								
W																								
T																								
F																								
S																								

Notes:

_____

_____

Week of: _____

Anxiety Level

	S	M	T	W	T	F	S
High							
Medium							
Low							
None							

Exercise

	S	M	T	W	T	F	S
AM							
Midday							
PM							

Sleep Tracker

	7	8	9	10	11	12	1	2	3	4	5	6	7	8	9	10	11	12	1	2	3	4	5	6
S																								
M																								
T																								
W																								
T																								
F																								
S																								

Other Symptoms	S	M	T	W	T	F	S

Daily Tracker

S	M	T	W	T	F	S

What I Ate Today

Appetite ⬆ or ⬇ Today?

Breakfast	Lunch	Dinner
Snack	**Snack**	**Snack**

Mood	Water
🙂 🙁 😕 😐 😠	◊◊◊◊◊◊◊◊

Weather

Notes

Where does it hurt?

Weight:

_____

Daily Tracker

S M T W T F S

What I Ate Today

Appetite ⬆ or ⬇ Today?

Breakfast	Lunch	Dinner
Snack	Snack	Snack

Mood	Water
🙂 🙁 😕 😐 😠	◊ ◊ ◊ ◊ ◊ ◊ ◊ ◊

Weather

Notes

Where does it hurt?

Weight:

_____

Daily Tracker

S M T W T F S

What I Ate Today

Appetite ⬆ or ⬇ Today?

Breakfast	Lunch	Dinner
Snack	Snack	Snack

Mood	Water
🙂 🙁 😕 😐 😠	💧💧💧💧💧💧💧💧

Where does it hurt?

Weather

Notes

Weight:

_____

Daily Tracker

S	M	T	W	T	F	S

What I Ate Today

Appetite ⬆ or ⬇ Today?

Breakfast	Lunch	Dinner
Snack	Snack	Snack

Mood	Water
☺ 🙁 😕 😐 😠	◊◊◊◊◊◊◊◊

Where does it hurt?

Weather

Notes

Weight:

_____

Daily Tracker

S M T W T F S

What I Ate Today		Appetite ⬆ or ⬇ Today?
Breakfast	Lunch	Dinner
Snack	Snack	Snack

Mood

☺ ☹ 😕 😐 😠

Water

◊ ◊ ◊ ◊ ◊ ◊ ◊ ◊

Weather

Notes

Where does it hurt?

Weight:

_____

Daily Tracker

| S | M | T | W | T | F | S |

What I Ate Today

Appetite ⬆ or ⬇ Today?

Breakfast	Lunch	Dinner
Snack	Snack	Snack

Mood

☺ ☹ 😖 😐 😠

Water

◊ ◊ ◊ ◊ ◊ ◊ ◊ ◊

Where does it hurt?

Weather

Notes

Weight:

_____

Daily Tracker

| S | M | T | W | T | F | S |

What I Ate Today

Appetite ⬆ or ⬇ Today?

Breakfast	Lunch	Dinner
Snack	Snack	Snack

Mood	Water
☺ ☹ ☺ 😐 😠	🌢🌢🌢🌢🌢🌢🌢

Weather

Notes

Where does it hurt?

Weight:

_____

Week At A Glance

Abdominal Migraine

	1	2	3	4	5	6	7	8	9	10	11	12	13	14	15	16	17	18	19	20	21	22	23	24
S																								
M																								
T																								
W																								
T																								
F																								
S																								

Cyclic Vomiting

	1	2	3	4	5	6	7	8	9	10	11	12	13	14	15	16	17	18	19	20	21	22	23	24
S																								
M																								
T																								
W																								
T																								
F																								
S																								

Notes:

_____

_____

Week of: _____

Anxiety Level

	S	M	T	W	T	F	S
High							
Medium							
Low							
None							

Exercise

	S	M	T	W	T	F	S
AM							
Midday							
PM							

Sleep Tracker

	7	8	9	10	11	12	1	2	3	4	5	6	7	8	9	10	11	12	1	2	3	4	5	6
S																								
M																								
T																								
W																								
T																								
F																								
S																								

Other Symptoms	S	M	T	W	T	F	S

Daily Tracker

S M T W T F S

What I Ate Today

Appetite ⬆ or ⬇ Today?

Breakfast	Lunch	Dinner
Snack	Snack	Snack

Mood	Water
☺ ☹ ☺ 😐 😠	🜄🜄🜄🜄🜄🜄🜄🜄

Weather

Notes

Where does it hurt?

Weight:

_____

Daily Tracker

S M T W T F S

What I Ate Today

Appetite ⬆ or ⬇ Today?

Breakfast	Lunch	Dinner
Snack	Snack	Snack

Mood	Water
🙂 🙁 😕 😐 😠	◊◊◊◊◊◊◊◊

Weather

Notes

Where does it hurt?

Weight:

_____

Daily Tracker

| S | M | T | W | T | F | S |

What I Ate Today

Appetite ⬆ or ⬇ Today?

Breakfast	Lunch	Dinner
Snack	Snack	Snack

Mood

☺ ☹ 😕 😐 😠

Water

◊ ◊ ◊ ◊ ◊ ◊ ◊ ◊

Weather

Notes

Where does it hurt?

Weight:

_____

Daily Tracker

S M T W T F S

What I Ate Today

Appetite ⬆ or ⬇ Today?

Breakfast	Lunch	Dinner
Snack	Snack	Snack

Mood

☺ ☹ 😕 😐 😠

Water

⬦⬦⬦⬦⬦⬦⬦⬦

Weather

Notes

Where does it hurt?

Weight:

_____

Daily Tracker

S M T W T F S

What I Ate Today

Appetite ⬆ or ⬇ Today?

Breakfast	Lunch	Dinner
Snack	Snack	Snack

Mood	Water
☺ ☹ ☺ ☺ ☹	◇◇◇◇◇◇◇◇

Weather

Notes

Where does it hurt?

Weight:

_____

Daily Tracker

| S | M | T | W | T | F | S |

What I Ate Today

Appetite ⬆ or ⬇ Today?

Breakfast	Lunch	Dinner
Snack	**Snack**	**Snack**

Mood

😊 ☹️ 😕 😐 😠

Water

◊ ◊ ◊ ◊ ◊ ◊ ◊ ◊

Where does it hurt?

Weather

Notes

Weight:

_____

Daily Tracker

S M T W T F S

What I Ate Today

Appetite ⬆ or ⬇ Today?

Breakfast	Lunch	Dinner
Snack	Snack	Snack

Mood

☺ ☹ 😕 😐 😠

Water

◊ ◊ ◊ ◊ ◊ ◊ ◊ ◊

Weather

Notes

Where does it hurt?

Weight:

_____

Week At A Glance

Abdominal Migraine

	1	2	3	4	5	6	7	8	9	10	11	12	13	14	15	16	17	18	19	20	21	22	23	24
S																								
M																								
T																								
W																								
T																								
F																								
S																								

Cyclic Vomiting

	1	2	3	4	5	6	7	8	9	10	11	12	13	14	15	16	17	18	19	20	21	22	23	24
S																								
M																								
T																								
W																								
T																								
F																								
S																								

Notes:

_____

_____

Week of: _____

Anxiety Level

	S	M	T	W	T	F	S
High							
Medium							
Low							
None							

Exercise

	S	M	T	W	T	F	S
AM							
Midday							
PM							

Sleep Tracker

	7	8	9	10	11	12	1	2	3	4	5	6	7	8	9	10	11	12	1	2	3	4	5	6
S																								
M																								
T																								
W																								
T																								
F																								
S																								

Other Symptoms	S	M	T	W	T	F	S

Daily Tracker

| S | M | T | W | T | F | S |

What I Ate Today

Appetite ⬆ or ⬇ Today?

Breakfast	Lunch	Dinner
Snack	Snack	Snack

Mood	Water
☺ ☹ ☺ ☺ ☹	◌◌◌◌◌◌◌◌

Weather

Notes

Where does it hurt?

Weight:

_____

Daily Tracker

S M T W T F S

What I Ate Today

Appetite ⬆ or ⬇ Today?

Breakfast	Lunch	Dinner
Snack	Snack	Snack

Mood

🙂 🙁 😕 😐 😠

Water

💧💧💧💧💧💧💧💧

Where does it hurt?

Weather

Notes

Weight:

_____

Daily Tracker

S M T W T F S

What I Ate Today		Appetite ⬆ or ⬇ Today?
Breakfast	Lunch	Dinner
Snack	Snack	Snack

Mood

☺ ☹ ☺ 😐 😠

Water

◊◊◊◊◊◊◊◊◊

Weather

Notes

Where does it hurt?

Weight:

_____

Daily Tracker

S M T W T F S

What I Ate Today		Appetite ⬆ or ⬇ Today?
Breakfast	Lunch	Dinner
Snack	Snack	Snack

Mood

☺ ☹ 😕 😐 😠

Water

◊ ◊ ◊ ◊ ◊ ◊ ◊ ◊

Weather

Notes

Where does it hurt?

Weight: _____

Daily Tracker

| S | M | T | W | T | F | S |

What I Ate Today

Appetite ⬆ or ⬇ Today?

Breakfast	Lunch	Dinner
Snack	Snack	Snack

Mood

😊 🙁 😕 😐 😠

Water

◊ ◊ ◊ ◊ ◊ ◊ ◊ ◊

Weather

Notes

Where does it hurt?

Weight:

_____

Daily Tracker

S M T W T F S

What I Ate Today

Appetite ⬆ or ⬇ Today?

Breakfast	Lunch	Dinner
Snack	Snack	Snack

Mood

😊 ☹️ 😟 😐 😠

Water

💧💧💧💧💧💧💧💧

Where does it hurt?

Weather

Notes

Weight:

_____

Daily Tracker

S M T W T F S

What I Ate Today

Appetite ⬆ or ⬇ Today?

Breakfast	Lunch	Dinner
Snack	Snack	Snack

Mood

😊 ☹️ 😕 😐 😣

Water

💧💧💧💧💧💧💧💧

Weather

Notes

Where does it hurt?

Weight: _____

Week At A Glance

Abdominal Migraine

	1	2	3	4	5	6	7	8	9	10	11	12	13	14	15	16	17	18	19	20	21	22	23	24
S																								
M																								
T																								
W																								
T																								
F																								
S																								

Cyclic Vomiting

	1	2	3	4	5	6	7	8	9	10	11	12	13	14	15	16	17	18	19	20	21	22	23	24
S																								
M																								
T																								
W																								
T																								
F																								
S																								

Notes:

_____

_____

Week of: _____

Anxiety Level

	S	M	T	W	T	F	S
High							
Medium							
Low							
None							

Exercise

	S	M	T	W	T	F	S
AM							
Midday							
PM							

Sleep Tracker

	7	8	9	10	11	12	1	2	3	4	5	6	7	8	9	10	11	12	1	2	3	4	5	6
S																								
M																								
T																								
W																								
T																								
F																								
S																								

Other Symptoms	S	M	T	W	T	F	S

Daily Tracker

S M T W T F S

What I Ate Today

Appetite ⬆ or ⬇ Today?

Breakfast	Lunch	Dinner
Snack	Snack	Snack

Mood

😊 😞 😐 😑 😠

Water

⬡⬡⬡⬡⬡⬡⬡⬡

Weather

Notes

Where does it hurt?

Weight:

_____

Daily Tracker

| S | M | T | W | T | F | S |

What I Ate Today

Appetite ⬆ or ⬇ Today?

Breakfast	Lunch	Dinner
Snack	Snack	Snack

Mood

😊 😟 😣 😑 😠

Water

💧💧💧💧💧💧💧💧

Weather

Notes

Where does it hurt?

Weight: _____

Daily Tracker

S M T W T F S

What I Ate Today

Appetite ⬆ or ⬇ Today?

Breakfast	Lunch	Dinner
Snack	Snack	Snack

Mood	Water
☺ ☹ ☺ 😐 😣	◊◊◊◊◊◊◊◊

Weather

Notes

Where does it hurt?

Weight:

_____

Daily Tracker

S M T W T F S

What I Ate Today

Appetite ⬆ or ⬇ Today?

Breakfast	Lunch	Dinner
Snack	Snack	Snack

Mood

🙂 🙁 😕 😐 😠

Water

💧💧💧💧💧💧💧💧

Weather

Notes

Where does it hurt?

Weight:

_____

Daily Tracker

S M T W T F S

What I Ate Today

Appetite ⬆ or ⬇ Today?

Breakfast	Lunch	Dinner
Snack	Snack	Snack

Mood

😊 😞 😐 😑 😠

Water

🜄 🜄 🜄 🜄 🜄 🜄 🜄 🜄

Weather

Notes

Where does it hurt?

Weight:

_____

Daily Tracker

| S | M | T | W | T | F | S |

What I Ate Today

Appetite ⬆ or ⬇ Today?

Breakfast	Lunch	Dinner
Snack	Snack	Snack

Mood

🙂 🙁 😕 😐 😠

Water

◊ ◊ ◊ ◊ ◊ ◊ ◊ ◊

Weather

Notes

Where does it hurt?

Weight:

_____

Daily Tracker

S	M	T	W	T	F	S

What I Ate Today

Appetite ⬆ or ⬇ Today?

Breakfast	Lunch	Dinner
Snack	Snack	Snack

Mood	Water
🙂 😟 😕 😐 😣	〇〇〇〇〇〇〇〇

Weather

Notes

Where does it hurt?

Weight:

_____

Week At A Glance

Abdominal Migraine

	1	2	3	4	5	6	7	8	9	10	11	12	13	14	15	16	17	18	19	20	21	22	23	24
S																								
M																								
T																								
W																								
T																								
F																								
S																								

Cyclic Vomiting

	1	2	3	4	5	6	7	8	9	10	11	12	13	14	15	16	17	18	19	20	21	22	23	24
S																								
M																								
T																								
W																								
T																								
F																								
S																								

Notes:

_____

_____

Week of: _____

Anxiety Level

	S	M	T	W	T	F	S
High							
Medium							
Low							
None							

Exercise

	S	M	T	W	T	F	S
AM							
Midday							
PM							

Sleep Tracker

	7	8	9	10	11	12	1	2	3	4	5	6	7	8	9	10	11	12	1	2	3	4	5	6
S																								
M																								
T																								
W																								
T																								
F																								
S																								

Other Symptoms	S	M	T	W	T	F	S

Daily Tracker

S M T W T F S

What I Ate Today

Appetite ⬆ or ⬇ Today?

Breakfast	Lunch	Dinner
Snack	Snack	Snack

Mood	Water
☺ ☹ ☺ ☺ ☹	◊◊◊◊◊◊◊◊

Weather

Notes

Where does it hurt?

Weight:

_____

Daily Tracker

S M T W T F S

What I Ate Today

Appetite ⬆ or ⬇ Today?

Breakfast	Lunch	Dinner
Snack	Snack	Snack

Mood	Water
☺ ☹ 😕 😐 😠	◊◊◊◊◊◊◊◊

Weather

Notes

Where does it hurt?

Weight:

_____

Daily Tracker

| S | M | T | W | T | F | S |

What I Ate Today

Appetite ⬆ or ⬇ Today?

Breakfast	Lunch	Dinner
Snack	Snack	Snack

Mood	Water
😊 ☹ 😕 😐 😠	💧💧💧💧💧💧💧💧

Where does it hurt?

Weather

Notes

Weight:

_____

Daily Tracker

| S | M | T | W | T | F | S |

What I Ate Today

Appetite ⬆ or ⬇ Today?

Breakfast	Lunch	Dinner
Snack	Snack	Snack

Mood

☺ ☹ 😐 😑 😠

Water

◇◇◇◇◇◇◇◇

Where does it hurt?

Weather

Notes

Weight:

_____

Daily Tracker

| S | M | T | W | T | F | S |

What I Ate Today

Appetite ⬆ or ⬇ Today?

Breakfast	Lunch	Dinner
Snack	Snack	Snack

Mood

🙂 🙁 😟 😐 😠

Water

◊ ◊ ◊ ◊ ◊ ◊ ◊ ◊

Weather

Notes

Where does it hurt?

Weight: _____

Daily Tracker

S M T W T F S

What I Ate Today

Appetite ⬆ or ⬇ Today?

Breakfast	Lunch	Dinner
Snack	Snack	Snack

Mood	Water
🙂 🙁 😕 😐 😠	💧💧💧💧💧💧💧💧

Weather

Notes

Where does it hurt?

Weight:

_____

Daily Tracker

S M T W T F S

What I Ate Today

Appetite ⬆ or ⬇ Today?

Breakfast	Lunch	Dinner
Snack	Snack	Snack

Mood

😊 🙁 😕 😐 😠

Water

◊ ◊ ◊ ◊ ◊ ◊ ◊ ◊

Weather

Notes

Where does it hurt?

Weight:

_____

Week At A Glance

Abdominal Migraine

	1	2	3	4	5	6	7	8	9	10	11	12	13	14	15	16	17	18	19	20	21	22	23	24
S																								
M																								
T																								
W																								
T																								
F																								
S																								

Cyclic Vomiting

	1	2	3	4	5	6	7	8	9	10	11	12	13	14	15	16	17	18	19	20	21	22	23	24
S																								
M																								
T																								
W																								
T																								
F																								
S																								

Notes:

_____

_____

Week of: _____

Anxiety Level

	S	M	T	W	T	F	S
High							
Medium							
Low							
None							

Exercise

	S	M	T	W	T	F	S
AM							
Midday							
PM							

Sleep Tracker

	7	8	9	10	11	12	1	2	3	4	5	6	7	8	9	10	11	12	1	2	3	4	5	6
S																								
M																								
T																								
W																								
T																								
F																								
S																								

Other Symptoms	S	M	T	W	T	F	S

Daily Tracker

S M T W T F S

What I Ate Today

Appetite ⬆ or ⬇ Today?

Breakfast	Lunch	Dinner
Snack	Snack	Snack

Mood

😊 😕 😟 😑 😣

Water

💧💧💧💧💧💧💧💧

Weather

Notes

Where does it hurt?

Weight:

_____

Daily Tracker

S M T W T F S

What I Ate Today

Appetite ⬆ or ⬇ Today?

Breakfast	Lunch	Dinner
Snack	Snack	Snack

Mood

☺ ☹ 😕 😐 😠

Water

⬭ ⬭ ⬭ ⬭ ⬭ ⬭ ⬭ ⬭

Weather

Notes

Where does it hurt?

Weight:

_____

Daily Tracker

S M T W T F S

What I Ate Today

Appetite ⬆ or ⬇ Today?

Breakfast	Lunch	Dinner
Snack	Snack	Snack

Mood

🙂 🙁 😕 😐 😠

Water

◊ ◊ ◊ ◊ ◊ ◊ ◊ ◊

Weather

Notes

Where does it hurt?

Weight:

_____

Daily Tracker

S M T W T F S

What I Ate Today

Appetite ⬆ or ⬇ Today?

Breakfast	Lunch	Dinner
Snack	Snack	Snack

Mood

😊 🙁 😕 😐 😠

Water

◇◇◇◇◇◇◇◇◇

Where does it hurt?

Weather

Notes

Weight:

_____

Daily Tracker

S   M   T   W   T   F   S

What I Ate Today

Appetite ⬆ or ⬇ Today?

Breakfast	Lunch	Dinner
Snack	Snack	Snack

Mood

🙂 🙁 😕 😐 😠

Water

◊ ◊ ◊ ◊ ◊ ◊ ◊ ◊

Weather

Notes

Where does it hurt?

Weight:

_____

Daily Tracker

S M T W T F S

What I Ate Today

Appetite ⬆ or ⬇ Today?

Breakfast	Lunch	Dinner
Snack	Snack	Snack

Mood

☺ ☹ 😕 😐 😠

Water

◊ ◊ ◊ ◊ ◊ ◊ ◊ ◊

Where does it hurt?

Weather

Notes

Weight:

_____

Daily Tracker

| S | M | T | W | T | F | S |

What I Ate Today

Appetite ⬆ or ⬇ Today?

Breakfast	Lunch	Dinner
Snack	Snack	Snack

Mood

😊 😞 😣 😐 😠

Water

🜄 🜄 🜄 🜄 🜄 🜄 🜄 🜄

Weather

Notes

Where does it hurt?

Weight:

_____

Week At A Glance

Abdominal Migraine

	1	2	3	4	5	6	7	8	9	10	11	12	13	14	15	16	17	18	19	20	21	22	23	24
S																								
M																								
T																								
W																								
T																								
F																								
S																								

Cyclic Vomiting

	1	2	3	4	5	6	7	8	9	10	11	12	13	14	15	16	17	18	19	20	21	22	23	24
S																								
M																								
T																								
W																								
T																								
F																								
S																								

Notes:

_____

_____

Week of: _____

Anxiety Level

	S	M	T	W	T	F	S
High							
Medium							
Low							
None							

Exercise

	S	M	T	W	T	F	S
AM							
Midday							
PM							

Sleep Tracker

	7	8	9	10	11	12	1	2	3	4	5	6	7	8	9	10	11	12	1	2	3	4	5	6
S																								
M																								
T																								
W																								
T																								
F																								
S																								

Other Symptoms	S	M	T	W	T	F	S

Daily Tracker

S M T W T F S

What I Ate Today

Appetite ⬆ or ⬇ Today?

Breakfast	Lunch	Dinner
Snack	Snack	Snack

Mood	Water
🙂 🙁 😕 😐 😠	◊ ◊ ◊ ◊ ◊ ◊ ◊ ◊

Weather

Notes

Where does it hurt?

Weight:

_____

Daily Tracker

S	M	T	W	T	F	S

What I Ate Today

Appetite ⬆ or ⬇ Today?

Breakfast	Lunch	Dinner
Snack	Snack	Snack

Mood

☺ ☹ 😕 😐 😠

Water

◊◊◊◊◊◊◊◊

Where does it hurt?

Weather

Notes

Weight:

_____

Daily Tracker

S M T W T F S

Breakfast	Lunch	Dinner
Snack	Snack	Snack

What I Ate Today

Appetite ⬆ or ⬇ Today?

Mood

😊 😞 😣 😐 😠

Water

◇◇◇◇◇◇◇◇

Weather

Notes

Where does it hurt?

Weight:

_____

Daily Tracker

| S | M | T | W | T | F | S |

What I Ate Today

Appetite ⬆ or ⬇ Today?

Breakfast	Lunch	Dinner
Snack	Snack	Snack

Mood

😊 🙁 😕 😐 😠

Water

💧💧💧💧💧💧💧💧

Where does it hurt?

Weather

Notes

Weight:

_____

Daily Tracker

| S | M | T | W | T | F | S |

What I Ate Today

Appetite ⬆ or ⬇ Today?

Breakfast	Lunch	Dinner
Snack	Snack	Snack

Mood	Water
😊 ☹ 😟 😐 😠	◊◊◊◊◊◊◊◊

Where does it hurt?

Weather

Notes

Weight:

_____

Daily Tracker

S M T W T F S

What I Ate Today

Appetite ⬆ or ⬇ Today?

Breakfast	Lunch	Dinner
Snack	Snack	Snack

Mood

🙂 🙁 😣 😐 😠

Water

◊◊◊◊◊◊◊◊

Weather

Notes

Where does it hurt?

Weight:

_____

Daily Tracker

S	M	T	W	T	F	S

What I Ate Today

Appetite ⬆ or ⬇ Today?

Breakfast	Lunch	Dinner
Snack	Snack	Snack

Mood

😊 😞 😐 😑 😠

Water

💧💧💧💧💧💧💧💧

Weather

Notes

Where does it hurt?

Weight:

_____

Week At A Glance

Abdominal Migraine

	1	2	3	4	5	6	7	8	9	10	11	12	13	14	15	16	17	18	19	20	21	22	23	24
S																								
M																								
T																								
W																								
T																								
F																								
S																								

Cyclic Vomiting

	1	2	3	4	5	6	7	8	9	10	11	12	13	14	15	16	17	18	19	20	21	22	23	24
S																								
M																								
T																								
W																								
T																								
F																								
S																								

Notes:

_____

_____

Week of: _____

Anxiety Level

	S	M	T	W	T	F	S
High							
Medium							
Low							
None							

Exercise

	S	M	T	W	T	F	S
AM							
Midday							
PM							

Sleep Tracker

	7	8	9	10	11	12	1	2	3	4	5	6	7	8	9	10	11	12	1	2	3	4	5	6
S																								
M																								
T																								
W																								
T																								
F																								
S																								

Other Symptoms	S	M	T	W	T	F	S

Daily Tracker

S M T W T F S

What I Ate Today

Appetite ⬆ or ⬇ Today?

Breakfast	Lunch	Dinner
Snack	Snack	Snack

Mood

☺ ☹ ☺ 😐 😠

Water

◌ ◌ ◌ ◌ ◌ ◌ ◌ ◌

Weather

Notes

Where does it hurt?

Weight:

_____

Daily Tracker

| S | M | T | W | T | F | S |

What I Ate Today

Appetite ⬆ or ⬇ Today?

Breakfast	Lunch	Dinner
Snack	Snack	Snack

Mood

😊 🙁 😕 😐 😠

Water

◊ ◊ ◊ ◊ ◊ ◊ ◊ ◊

Weather

Notes

Where does it hurt?

Weight: _____

Daily Tracker

S M T W T F S

What I Ate Today

Appetite ⬆ or ⬇ Today?

Breakfast	Lunch	Dinner
Snack	Snack	Snack

Mood

☺ ☹ 😐 😑 😠

Water

◊◊◊◊◊◊◊◊

Weather

Notes

Where does it hurt?

Weight:

_____

Daily Tracker

S	M	T	W	T	F	S

What I Ate Today

Appetite ⬆ or ⬇ Today?

Breakfast	Lunch	Dinner
Snack	Snack	Snack

Mood	Water
🙂 🙁 😕 😐 😠	◊◊◊◊◊◊◊◊

Where does it hurt?

Weather

Notes

Weight: _____

Daily Tracker

S M T W T F S

What I Ate Today

Appetite ⬆ or ⬇ Today?

Breakfast	Lunch	Dinner
Snack	Snack	Snack

Mood

☺ ☹ 😐 😑 😠

Water

◊ ◊ ◊ ◊ ◊ ◊ ◊ ◊

Weather

Notes

Where does it hurt?

Weight: _____

Daily Tracker

| S | M | T | W | T | F | S |

What I Ate Today

Appetite ⬆ or ⬇ Today?

Breakfast	Lunch	Dinner
Snack	Snack	Snack

Mood

☺ ☹ ☹ 😐 😠

Water

◊◊◊◊◊◊◊◊

Weather

Notes

Where does it hurt?

Weight:

_____

Daily Tracker

S	M	T	W	T	F	S

What I Ate Today		Appetite ⬆ or ⬇ Today?
Breakfast	**Lunch**	**Dinner**
Snack	**Snack**	**Snack**

Mood	Water
🙂 🙁 😕 😐 😠	◊◊◊◊◊◊◊◊

Weather

Notes

Where does it hurt?

Weight: _____

Week At A Glance

Abdominal Migraine

	1	2	3	4	5	6	7	8	9	10	11	12	13	14	15	16	17	18	19	20	21	22	23	24
S																								
M																								
T																								
W																								
T																								
F																								
S																								

Cyclic Vomiting

	1	2	3	4	5	6	7	8	9	10	11	12	13	14	15	16	17	18	19	20	21	22	23	24
S																								
M																								
T																								
W																								
T																								
F																								
S																								

Notes:

_____

_____

Week of: _____

Anxiety Level

	S	M	T	W	T	F	S
High							
Medium							
Low							
None							

Exercise

	S	M	T	W	T	F	S
AM							
Midday							
PM							

Sleep Tracker

	7	8	9	10	11	12	1	2	3	4	5	6	7	8	9	10	11	12	1	2	3	4	5	6
S																								
M																								
T																								
W																								
T																								
F																								
S																								

Other Symptoms	S	M	T	W	T	F	S

Daily Tracker

S M T W T F S

What I Ate Today

Appetite ⬆ or ⬇ Today?

Breakfast	Lunch	Dinner
Snack	Snack	Snack

Mood	Water
☺ ☹ ☺ ☺ ☹	◊◊◊◊◊◊◊◊

Weather

Notes

Where does it hurt?

Weight:

_____

Daily Tracker

S M T W T F S

What I Ate Today

Appetite ⬆ or ⬇ Today?

Breakfast	Lunch	Dinner
Snack	Snack	Snack

Mood

🙂 🙁 😕 😐 😠

Water

◇◇◇◇◇◇◇◇

Where does it hurt?

Weather

Notes

Weight:

_____

Daily Tracker

S M T W T F S

What I Ate Today

Appetite ⬆ or ⬇ Today?

Breakfast	Lunch	Dinner
Snack	Snack	Snack

Mood	Water
☺ ☹ ☺ ☺ ☹	◊◊◊◊◊◊◊◊

Where does it hurt?

Weather

Notes

Weight:

_____

Daily Tracker

S M T W T F S

What I Ate Today

Appetite ⬆ or ⬇ Today?

Breakfast	Lunch	Dinner
Snack	Snack	Snack

Mood	Water
☺ ☹ ☹ 😐 😠	◊◊◊◊◊◊◊◊

Weather

Notes

Where does it hurt?

Weight:

_____

Daily Tracker

| S | M | T | W | T | F | S |

What I Ate Today

Appetite ⬆ or ⬇ Today?

Breakfast	Lunch	Dinner
Snack	Snack	Snack

Mood	Water
☺ ☹ ☹ 😐 😠	◊◊◊◊◊◊◊◊

Weather

Notes

Where does it hurt?

Weight:

_____

Daily Tracker

S M T W T F S

What I Ate Today

Appetite ⬆ or ⬇ Today?

Breakfast	Lunch	Dinner
Snack	Snack	Snack

Mood

😊 😟 😕 😐 😠

Water

◇◇◇◇◇◇◇◇

Where does it hurt?

Weather

Notes

Weight:

_____

Daily Tracker

S M T W T F S

What I Ate Today

Appetite ⬆ or ⬇ Today?

Breakfast	Lunch	Dinner
Snack	Snack	Snack

Mood

😊 😞 😕 😐 😠

Water

◊ ◊ ◊ ◊ ◊ ◊ ◊ ◊

Weather

Notes

Where does it hurt?

Weight:

_____

Week At A Glance

Abdominal Migraine

	1	2	3	4	5	6	7	8	9	10	11	12	13	14	15	16	17	18	19	20	21	22	23	24
S																								
M																								
T																								
W																								
T																								
F																								
S																								

Cyclic Vomiting

	1	2	3	4	5	6	7	8	9	10	11	12	13	14	15	16	17	18	19	20	21	22	23	24
S																								
M																								
T																								
W																								
T																								
F																								
S																								

Notes:

_____

_____

Week of: _____

Anxiety Level							
	S	M	T	W	T	F	S
High							
Medium							
Low							
None							

Exercise							
	S	M	T	W	T	F	S
AM							
Midday							
PM							

Sleep Tracker																								
	7	8	9	10	11	12	1	2	3	4	5	6	7	8	9	10	11	12	1	2	3	4	5	6
S																								
M																								
T																								
W																								
T																								
F																								
S																								

Other Symptoms	S	M	T	W	T	F	S

Daily Tracker

S M T W T F S

What I Ate Today

Appetite ⬆ or ⬇ Today?

Breakfast	Lunch	Dinner
Snack	Snack	Snack

Mood

😊 ☹️ 😐 😑 😠

Water

💧💧💧💧💧💧💧💧

Where does it hurt?

Weather

Notes

Weight:

_____

Daily Tracker

| S | M | T | W | T | F | S |

What I Ate Today

Appetite ⬆ or ⬇ Today?

Breakfast	Lunch	Dinner
Snack	**Snack**	**Snack**

Mood

☺ ☹ ☺ 😐 😠

Water

◇◇◇◇◇◇◇◇

Where does it hurt?

Weather

Notes

Weight:

_____

Daily Tracker

S M T W T F S

What I Ate Today		Appetite ⬆ or ⬇ Today?
Breakfast	Lunch	Dinner
Snack	Snack	Snack

Mood

🙂 🙁 😕 😐 😣

Water

◇◇◇◇◇◇◇◇

Weather

Notes

Where does it hurt?

Weight: _____

Daily Tracker

S M T W T F S

What I Ate Today

Appetite ⬆ or ⬇ Today?

Breakfast	Lunch	Dinner
Snack	Snack	Snack

Mood	Water
🙂 ☹ 🙁 😐 😠	〇〇〇〇〇〇〇〇〇

Where does it hurt?

Weather

Notes

Weight:

_____

Daily Tracker

S M T W T F S

What I Ate Today		Appetite ⬆ or ⬇ Today?
Breakfast	**Lunch**	**Dinner**
Snack	**Snack**	**Snack**

Mood

☺ ☹ ☺ 😐 😠

Water

◇◇◇◇◇◇◇◇

Weather

Where does it hurt?

Notes

Weight:

_____

Daily Tracker

S M T W T F S

What I Ate Today

Appetite ⬆ or ⬇ Today?

Breakfast	Lunch	Dinner
Snack	Snack	Snack

Mood

😊 ☹ 😕 😐 😠

Water

◇◇◇◇◇◇◇◇

Where does it hurt?

Weather

Notes

Weight:

_____

Daily Tracker

S M T W T F S

What I Ate Today

Appetite ⬆ or ⬇ Today?

Breakfast	Lunch	Dinner
Snack	Snack	Snack

Mood

☺ ☹ 😐 😑 😠

Water

◇◇◇◇◇◇◇◇

Where does it hurt?

Weather

Notes

Weight:

_____

Week At A Glance

Abdominal Migraine

	1	2	3	4	5	6	7	8	9	10	11	12	13	14	15	16	17	18	19	20	21	22	23	24
S																								
M																								
T																								
W																								
T																								
F																								
S																								

Cyclic Vomiting

	1	2	3	4	5	6	7	8	9	10	11	12	13	14	15	16	17	18	19	20	21	22	23	24
S																								
M																								
T																								
W																								
T																								
F																								
S																								

Notes:

_____

_____

Week of: _____

Anxiety Level

	S	M	T	W	T	F	S
High							
Medium							
Low							
None							

Exercise

	S	M	T	W	T	F	S
AM							
Midday							
PM							

Sleep Tracker

	7	8	9	10	11	12	1	2	3	4	5	6	7	8	9	10	11	12	1	2	3	4	5	6
S																								
M																								
T																								
W																								
T																								
F																								
S																								

Other Symptoms	S	M	T	W	T	F	S

Daily Tracker

| S | M | T | W | T | F | S |

What I Ate Today

Appetite ⬆ or ⬇ Today?

Breakfast	Lunch	Dinner
Snack	Snack	Snack

Mood

🙂 🙁 😐 😑 😠

Water

◊ ◊ ◊ ◊ ◊ ◊ ◊ ◊

Weather

Notes

Where does it hurt?

Weight:

_____

Daily Tracker

| S | M | T | W | T | F | S |

What I Ate Today

Appetite ⬆ or ⬇ Today?

Breakfast	Lunch	Dinner
Snack	Snack	Snack

Mood	Water
☺ ☹ 😕 😐 😠	〇〇〇〇〇〇〇〇

Weather

Notes

Where does it hurt?

Weight:

_____

Daily Tracker

S M T W T F S

What I Ate Today		Appetite ⬆ or ⬇ Today?
Breakfast	Lunch	Dinner
Snack	Snack	Snack

Mood

😊 😞 😟 😐 😠

Water

◇◇◇◇◇◇◇◇

Weather

Notes

Where does it hurt?

Weight:

_____

Daily Tracker

S M T W T F S

What I Ate Today

Appetite ⬆ or ⬇ Today?

Breakfast	Lunch	Dinner
Snack	Snack	Snack

Mood

☺ ☹ 😕 😐 😠

Water

◊ ◊ ◊ ◊ ◊ ◊ ◊ ◊

Where does it hurt?

Weather

Notes

Weight:

_____

Daily Tracker

S M T W T F S

What I Ate Today

Appetite ⬆ or ⬇ Today?

Breakfast	Lunch	Dinner
Snack	Snack	Snack

Mood

🙂 🙁 😕 😐 😣

Water

◊ ◊ ◊ ◊ ◊ ◊ ◊ ◊

Weather

Notes

Where does it hurt?

Weight:
_____

Daily Tracker

| S | M | T | W | T | F | S |

What I Ate Today   Appetite ⬆ or ⬇ Today?

Breakfast	Lunch	Dinner
Snack	Snack	Snack

Mood	Water
☺ ☹ ☹ 😐 😠	◊◊◊◊◊◊◊◊

Where does it hurt?

Weather

Notes

Weight:

_____

Daily Tracker

S M T W T F S

What I Ate Today		Appetite ⬆ or ⬇ Today?
Breakfast	Lunch	Dinner
Snack	Snack	Snack

Mood

☺ ☹ 😕 😐 😠

Water

⬡⬡⬡⬡⬡⬡⬡⬡⬡

Weather

Notes

Where does it hurt?

Weight:

_____

Week At A Glance

Abdominal Migraine

	1	2	3	4	5	6	7	8	9	10	11	12	13	14	15	16	17	18	19	20	21	22	23	24
S																								
M																								
T																								
W																								
T																								
F																								
S																								

Cyclic Vomiting

	1	2	3	4	5	6	7	8	9	10	11	12	13	14	15	16	17	18	19	20	21	22	23	24
S																								
M																								
T																								
W																								
T																								
F																								
S																								

Notes:

_____

_____

Week of: _____

Anxiety Level

	S	M	T	W	T	F	S
High							
Medium							
Low							
None							

Exercise

	S	M	T	W	T	F	S
AM							
Midday							
PM							

Sleep Tracker

	7	8	9	10	11	12	1	2	3	4	5	6	7	8	9	10	11	12	1	2	3	4	5	6
S																								
M																								
T																								
W																								
T																								
F																								
S																								

Other Symptoms	S	M	T	W	T	F	S

Daily Tracker

S M T W T F S

What I Ate Today

Appetite ⬆ or ⬇ Today?

Breakfast	Lunch	Dinner
Snack	Snack	Snack

Mood

😊 😞 😕 😐 😠

Water

◊◊◊◊◊◊◊◊

Weather

Notes

Where does it hurt?

Weight:

_____

Daily Tracker

S M T W T F S

What I Ate Today

Appetite ⬆ or ⬇ Today?

Breakfast	Lunch	Dinner
Snack	Snack	Snack

Mood	Water
☺ ☹ ☺ ☺ 😠	〇〇〇〇〇〇〇〇

Where does it hurt?

Weather

Notes

Weight:

_____

Daily Tracker

S M T W T F S

What I Ate Today

Appetite ⬆ or ⬇ Today?

Breakfast	Lunch	Dinner
Snack	Snack	Snack

Mood

😊 😟 🙁 😐 😠

Water

💧💧💧💧💧💧💧💧

Where does it hurt?

Weather

Notes

Weight:

_____

Daily Tracker

S M T W T F S

What I Ate Today

Appetite ⬆ or ⬇ Today?

Breakfast	Lunch	Dinner
Snack	Snack	Snack

Mood

🙂 🙁 😐 😑 😠

Water

◇◇◇◇◇◇◇◇◇

Where does it hurt?

Weather

Notes

Weight:

_____

Daily Tracker

| S | M | T | W | T | F | S |

What I Ate Today

Appetite ⬆ or ⬇ Today?

Breakfast	Lunch	Dinner
Snack	Snack	Snack

Mood

☺ ☹ 😕 😐 😠

Water

◊ ◊ ◊ ◊ ◊ ◊ ◊ ◊

Weather

Notes

Where does it hurt?

Weight:

_____

Daily Tracker

| S | M | T | W | T | F | S |

What I Ate Today

Appetite ⬆ or ⬇ Today?

Breakfast	Lunch	Dinner
Snack	Snack	Snack

Mood	Water
☺ ☹ ☹ 😐 😠	◇◇◇◇◇◇◇◇

Weather

Notes

Where does it hurt?

Weight:

_____

Daily Tracker

| S | M | T | W | T | F | S |

What I Ate Today

Appetite ⬆ or ⬇ Today?

Breakfast	Lunch	Dinner
Snack	Snack	Snack

Mood

☺ ☹ ☺ 😐 😠

Water

◇◇◇◇◇◇◇◇

Weather

Notes

Where does it hurt?

Weight:

_____

Made in United States
North Haven, CT
22 October 2022

25780438R00070